Safia Othmani
Hana Hedhli
Rim Ben Kaddour

ABCDE APPROACH: INPUT ON NURSING ASSESSMENT IN EMERGENCY DEPARTMENTS

Safia Othmani
Hana Hedhli
Rim Ben Kaddour

ABCDE APPROACH: INPUT ON NURSING ASSESSMENT IN EMERGENCY DEPARTMENTS

ScienciaScripts

Imprint

Any brand names and product names mentioned in this book are subject to trademark, brand or patent protection and are trademarks or registered trademarks of their respective holders. The use of brand names, product names, common names, trade names, product descriptions etc. even without a particular marking in this work is in no way to be construed to mean that such names may be regarded as unrestricted in respect of trademark and brand protection legislation and could thus be used by anyone.

Cover image: www.ingimage.com

This book is a translation from the original published under ISBN 978-620-3-42543-7.

Publisher:
Sciencia Scripts
is a trademark of
Dodo Books Indian Ocean Ltd., member of the OmniScriptum S.R.L Publishing group
str. A.Russo 15, of. 61, Chisinau-2068, Republic of Moldova Europe
Printed at: see last page
ISBN: 978-620-4-11376-0

Table of Contents

List Of Abbreviations

ABCDE: Airway, Breathing, Circulation, Disability, Exposure.

CHU : University Hospital Centre.

HCN: Hôpital Charles Nicoles.

HHT: Habib Thameur Hospital.

VAS: upper airway.

SpO2: Pulse Oxygen Saturation.

HR: heart rate.

BP: blood pressure.

GAD: Finger prick blood glucose.

ATLS: Advanced Trauma Life Support

WHO: World Health Organization

 ISP: firefighter nurse

COVID-19 :Coronavirus infection disease 2019

CGS: Coma Glasgow Score

Introduction

The emergency department must receive all the people who are referred to it or who come to it by ensuring that they are appropriately received and cared for according to their state of health. This reception and management aims to satisfy and inform these people as well as the various emergency department contacts, and is conditioned by a good initial clinical assessment. These clinical states are determined by the establishment of a systematic neurological, ventilatory and circulatory vital assessment. Major impairment of one of these 3 major functions will identify a patient as having a life-threatening emergency requiring immediate care [1]. However, in order to guarantee rapidity and continuity of care, it is essential to obtain the best possible "interpersonal" interaction in order to optimize the chain of survival and thus offer patients the maximum chance of surviving a critical situation. Therefore, the integration of such an approach as the ABCDE approach in the emergency room seems to be an ideal solution, due to its systematized nature, for the management of patients [2]. In general, the clinical signs of critical illness are similar regardless of the underlying process because they reflect failure of the respiratory, cardiovascular and neurological systems. And the measurement and recording of physiological parameters in critically ill patients is not performed as often as desired. Thus, the use of the ABCDE approach is interested in specifying the parameters of the following entities in a comprehensive manner:

AIRWAY: Airway clearance and cervical spine protection BREATHING: Assessment of breathing and ventilation CIRCULATION: Assessment of hemodynamic status
DISABILITY: Assessment of neurological status EXPOSURE: Environment and skin examination This approach allows for a rapid, exhaustive, standardized, prioritized assessment of vital distress in critically ill patients. This approach is

widely used in emergency departments, and as an integral part of the health care team, nurses must master this approach, which is of great value in daily practice. It seems to be a universal tool, usable by all health professionals, practical and reliable, reproducible, relevant in emergency care and situations at risk of decompensation, which would allow to improve the clinical evaluation of a patient, to establish a diagnosis sometimes, to treat a patient and to evaluate the effectiveness of the treatment and to communicate about the clinical situation of a patient. The emergency context is becoming more and more complex to deal with due to the difficulty in organizing the different situations in the training of caregivers. To do this, it is necessary to apply a modern, rapid and well-organized work method such as the ABCDE approach, which is an effective method for guiding the process of caring for emergency patients in the different sectors, especially in the emergency room. The patients who can benefit from it are numerous in traumatology as in other medical fields or others[3], and to apply this method well it is necessary to have qualified and trained personnel on this method and predisposing theoretical and practical knowledge. The main purpose of the study is to evaluate the knowledge of nurses working in emergency departments about the ABCDE approach and to find out if they think that this approach is a good tool for transmitting interpersonal information during inter-team communication. From this research question arose the idea of carrying out a quantitative descriptive study through a questionnaire to evaluate the knowledge of the ABCDE approach of the emergency nurses in order to promote the development of the use of this approach.

Materials and Methods

1. Type of study:

We conducted a descriptive cross-sectional multicenter study to collect the necessary data to achieve our work objective.

2. Presentation of the study method :

We conducted a quantitative descriptive research to evaluate the nurses' knowledge of the ABCDE approach in the management of critically ill patients in an emergency department, as well as the interest given by these nurses to the implementation of a common protocol.

3. Choice and construction of the survey tool :

The survey tool consists of a questionnaire addressed to emergency room nurses, structured according to the model attached.

The questionnaire was designed to be easy to use, with an estimated response time of about ten minutes, in order to increase the number of returns from nurses and minimize missing responses.

This questionnaire is composed of 19 questions. It is based on closed questions with binary answers "Yes/No" and multiple choice questions were divided into the following parts:

- Identification of the target population.

- The particularities of an emergency service.

- Nursing knowledge of the ABCDE approach.

- The value of implementing the ABCDE approach in the emergency room and its impact on the care process.

4. Selection of target location and population :

The study population targeted nurses working in emergency departments, since they are the focus of our study.

a. Inclusion criteria

- The nurses who were present during the survey during the different work sessions: morning, afternoon and night.
- Nurses who agreed to participate in the study.
- Emergency medical technicians.

b. Non-inclusion criteria

- Caregivers acting as nurses.

- Nurses on leave

c. Exclusion criteria

- Nurses who refused to participate in the study (non-consenting).

Our research was carried out multicentrically, at the level of the emergency ward of the Centre Hospitalo-universitaire (CHU) Charles Nicolle, La Rabta and Habib Thameur.

5. Conduct of the investigation :

The survey took place during the month of April 2020 until June 14, 2020. The results of the survey were analysed.

6. Data analysis :

The database was also processed by GOOGLE FORMS software, as well as GOOGLE spreadsheets and EXCEL software to produce tables, graphs and histograms.

Based on data from the literature,

7. Ethical considerations :

Based on the principle that every research must comply with certain ethical principles, our work was carried out in strict compliance with the provision relating to the principles, namely the respect of the freedom of participation of nurses in this survey envisaged for the collection of information. The respect of anonymity and confidentiality regarding the identity of the participants, during the final presentation of the results of the study.

Results

The results of our survey were analyzed among 65 nurses (N=65) who worked in the emergency departments of the 3 hospitals in Tunis.

She is interested in specifying data on:

- Socio-demographic and professional characteristics of the nurses questioned.

- The particularities of an emergency service.

- Nursing knowledge of the ABCDE approach

- The value of implementing the ABCDE approach in the emergency department

I. Identification of the study population :

1. Gender distribution of the sample :

Among the 65 nurses participating in this study, 29 were female, i.e. 44.6% with a sex ratio of 1.24 (Fig.1).

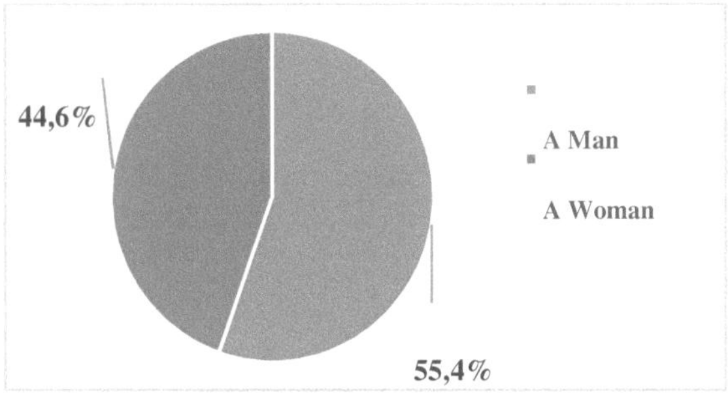

Fig.1: Distribution of the sample by gender

2. The distribution of the sample by education :

The participants questioned are represented by multipurpose nurses in 59 cases (90.8%) and emergency technicians in 9.2%. (Fig.2)

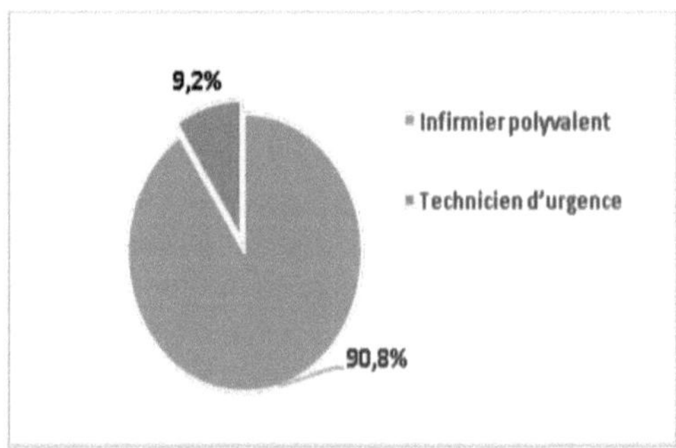

Fig.2: Distribution of the sample according to training.

3. The distribution of the sample by occupation :

It was found that 61 (93.8%) of the participants were bedside nurses.

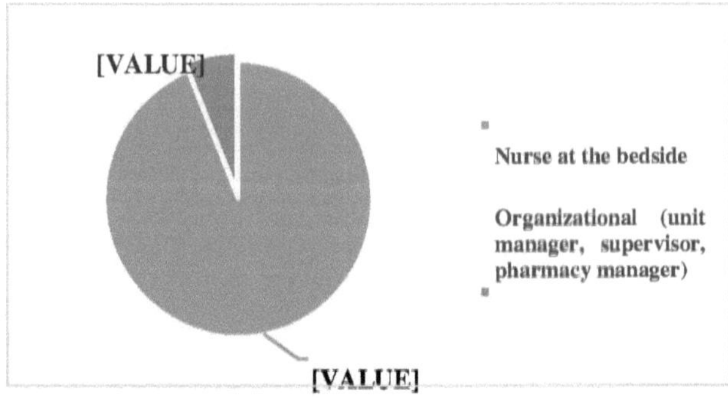

Fig.3: Distribution of the sample by occupation.

4. Distribution of the sample by age and seniority :

The analysis of the results showed that 56.9% of the participants were aged between 30 and 49 years. (Fig.4)

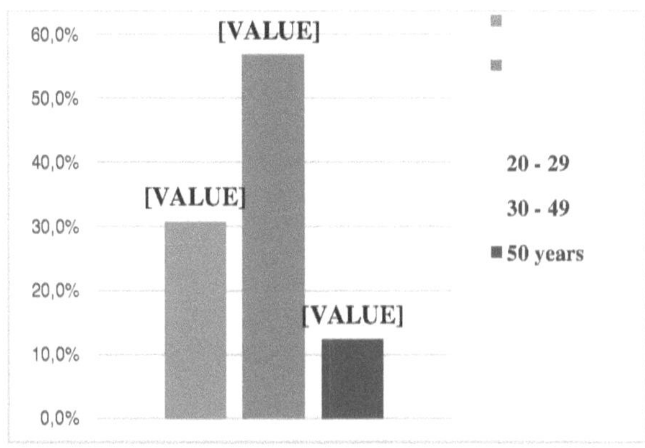

Fig.4: Age distribution of the sample.

Thirty-five nurses (53.8%) had less than or equal to 5 years of work experience. (Fig.5)

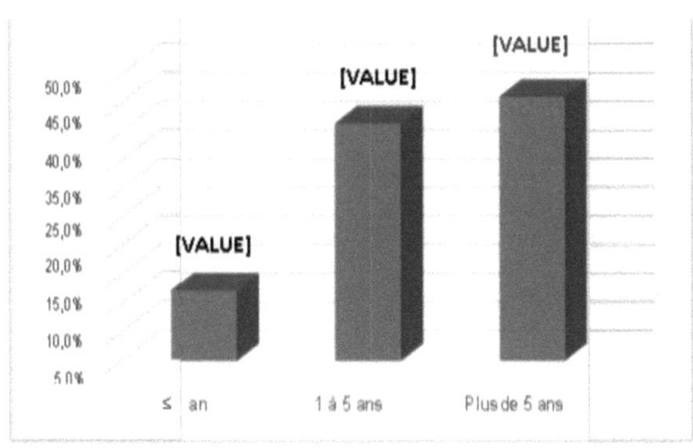

Fig.5: Distribution of participants according to seniority in the profession.

Regarding the length of time in the emergency department, we find that 44.6% of the participants had experience between 1 and 5 years. 43.1% had experience of more than 5 years. (Fig.6)

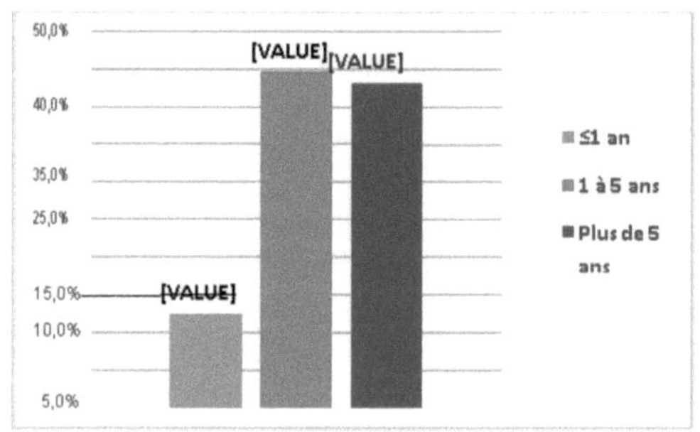

Fig.6: Distribution of the sample according to seniority in the emergency department.

5. The distribution of the sample according to participation in previous training :

Regarding participation in previous training on emergency care and first aid, 36 of the respondents (55.4%) had received training on emergency care and first aid. (Fig.7)

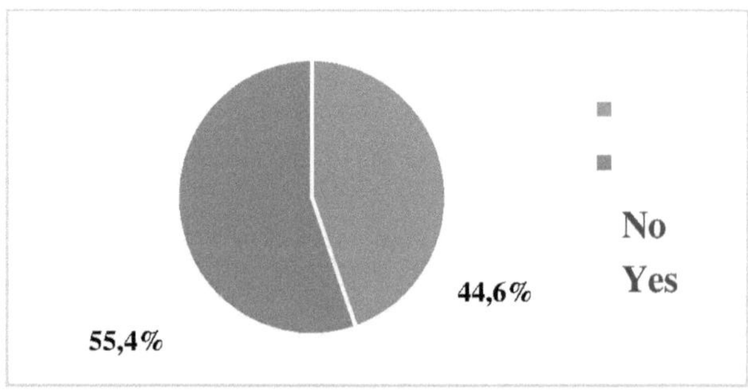

Fig.7: Participation in previous trainings.

The nurses who had previous training were distributed respectively and according to the hospital of exercise that it is HCN, Rabta and HT in 58%, 45% and 65%. (Fig.8)

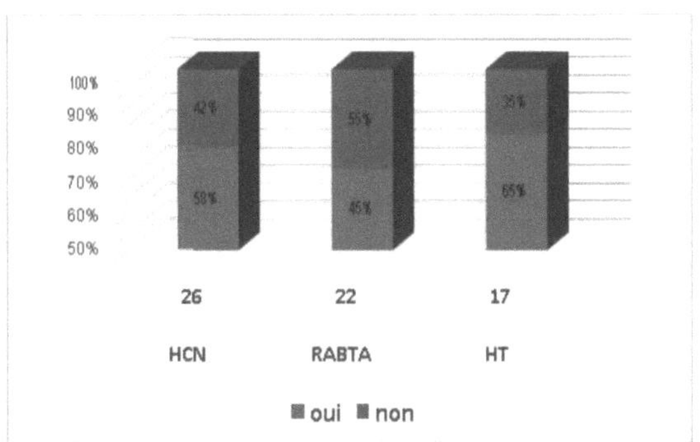

Fig.8: Distribution of previous training according to hospital of practice.

II. The particularity of an emergency service:

1. Protocolization of initial care in emergency departments :

It was found that 40 (61.5%) of the staff surveyed reported that the management of the disease was not protocolized in their departments. (Fig.9)

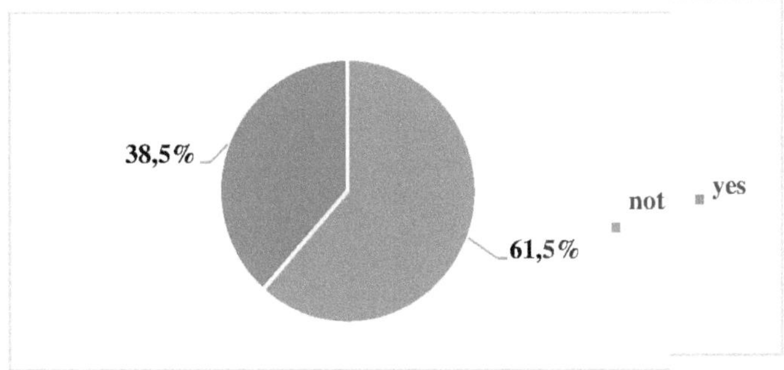

Fig.9 : Protocolisation of the initial care in the emergency room.

2. The impact of the implementation of a management protocol on interpersonal communication :

According to our study, 55 of the questioned caregivers (84.6%) affirmed that the implementation of a standardized management protocol will contribute to interpersonal and management improvement. (Fig.10) of communication

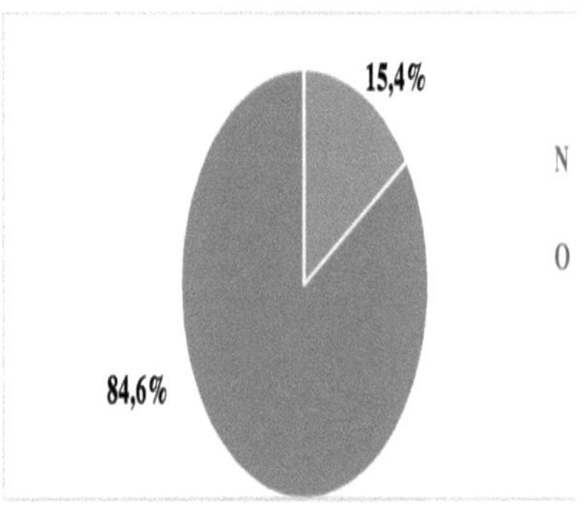

Fig.10: The impact of the implementation of a care protocol on interpersonal communication.

The nurses who answered that the implementation of such a protocol will facilitate the care and interpersonal communication were distributed respectively and according to the hospital of exercise HCN, Rabta and HHT in 85%, 82%, 88%. (Fig.11)

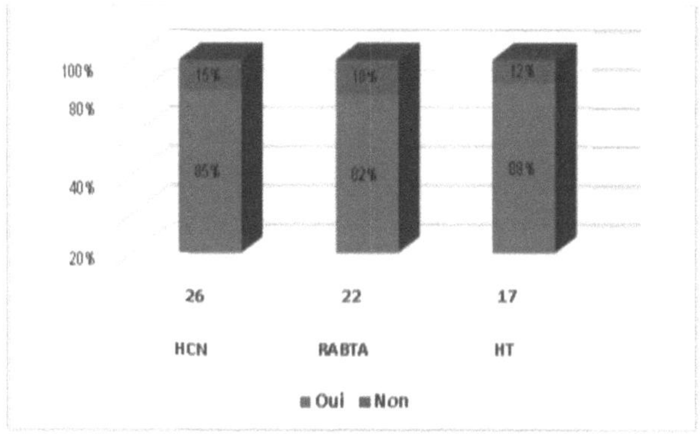

Fig.11: The impact of the implementation of a protocol by hospital.

III. Nursing knowledge on the ABCDE approach :

1.   Global knowledge of the ABCDE approach:

The analysis of the results on nursing knowledge of the ABCDE approach showed that 41 or 63.1% did not know that such an assessment approach exists. (Fig.12)

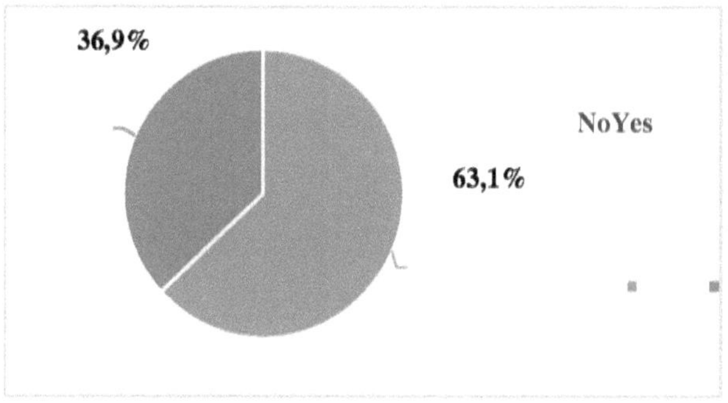

Fig.12: Knowledge of the ABCDE approach

2. The use of the ABCDE approach in daily practice :

Nine point two percent of participants used the ABCDE approach in daily practice. (Fig.13)

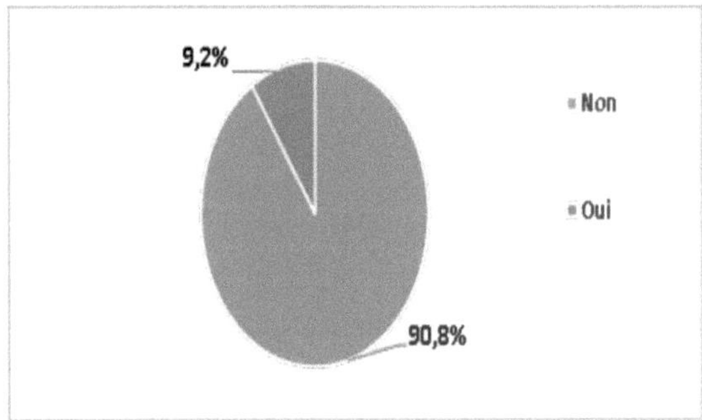

Fig.13: The use of the ABCDE approach in daily practice.

3. The overall characteristics of the ABCDE approach

Seventy-six percent of the respondents noted that it allows for speed in the initial assessment, while 88% of the cases recognized that it follows a certain chronology. (Fig.14)

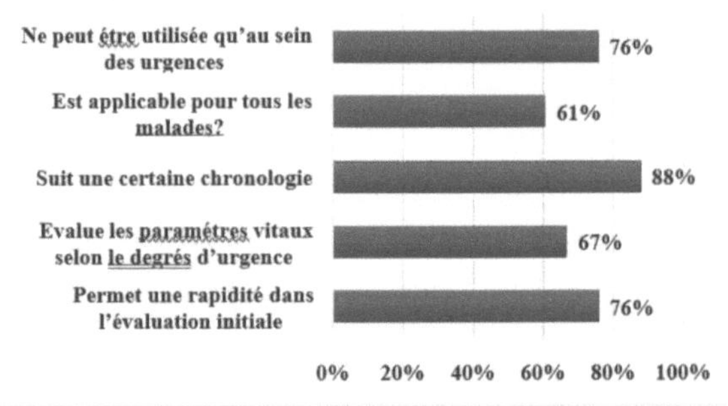

Fig.14: The overall characteristics of the ABCDE approach

4. Nurses' knowledge of Airway, Breathing, Circulation, Disability, Exposure :

• **Entity A "Airway"**: it was found that among the 65 nurses questioned, 13.8% recognized all of the items in this evaluation step.

\- 82% of respondents reported that it only assesses the risk of VAS obstruction, according to 46% of respondents it assesses the risk of inhalation.

\- 69% of the respondents recognized that the airway is at risk in case of consciousness disorder. (Fig.15)

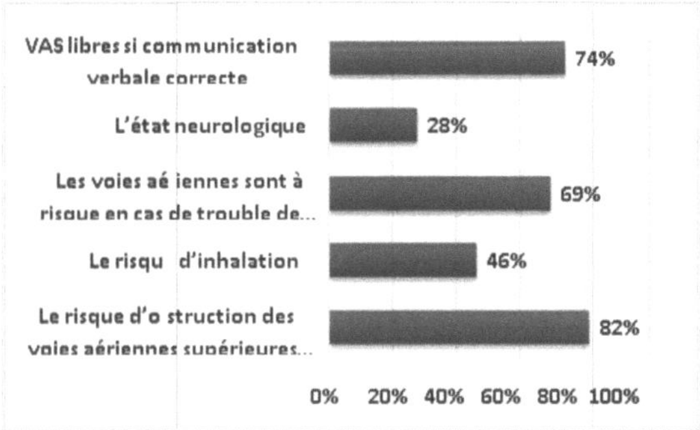

Fig.15 : Nursing knowledge on the entity A" Airway ".

•**Entity B "Breathing"**: it was found that 15.1% of the respondents parameters related to this entity. recognized all the

\- 94% of respondents noted that it consists of measuring respiratory SpO2. and 80% at the rate

\- 22% of the respondents reported that it assesses heart rate. (Fig.16)

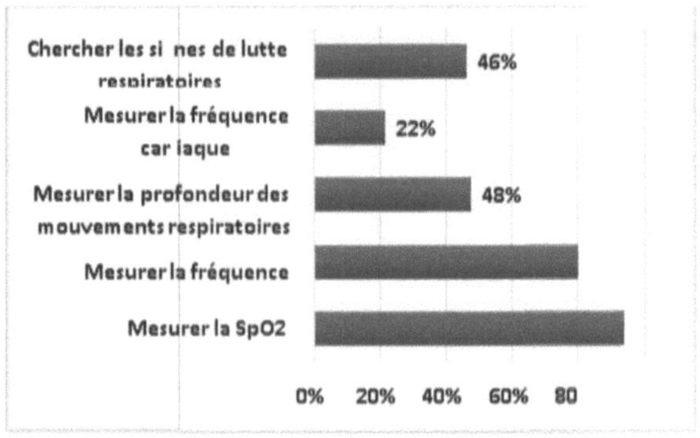

Fig.16 : Nursing knowledge on the entity "Breathing".

• **Entity C "Circulation"**: 38.5% of the participants mentioned all the parameters assessing the hemodynamic state.

- 97% of respondents limited themselves to measuring BP and HR, 80% to palpating peripheral and central pulses.

- 55% noted the verification of the colour and the warmth of the extremities. (Fig.17)

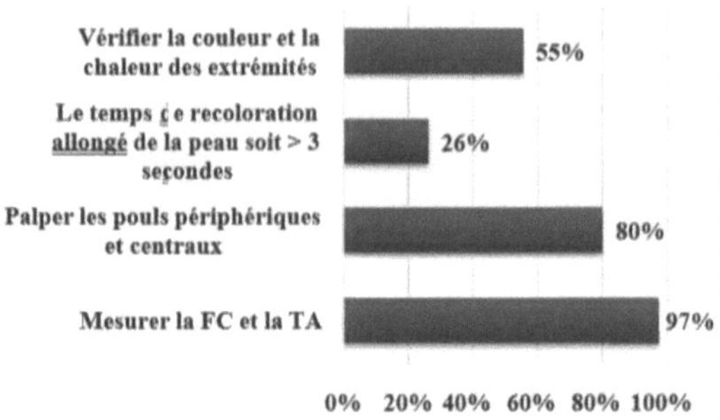

Fig.17 : Nursing knowledge on the assessment of the hemodynamic state

• **Entity D "Disability",** 16.9% of participants were found to have reported the appropriate items to this entity.

- 97% of respondents relied solely on the Glasgow Coma Scale (GCS) assessment.

- 66% mentioned the practice of DSM.

- 32% of respondents answered about the procedures used to assess neurological status and to identify signs of localization.

- 9% of evaluation respondents (Fig. 18) included radiological **exploration in this loop. radiology in this loop**

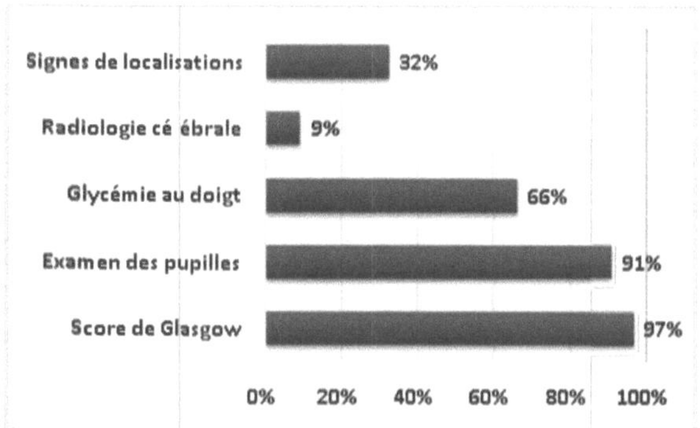

Fig.18 : Nursing knowledge on the entity "Disability

• Regarding the study of entity E "Exposure" it was found that 69.2% insisted on the need to do a skin examination to assess a patient.

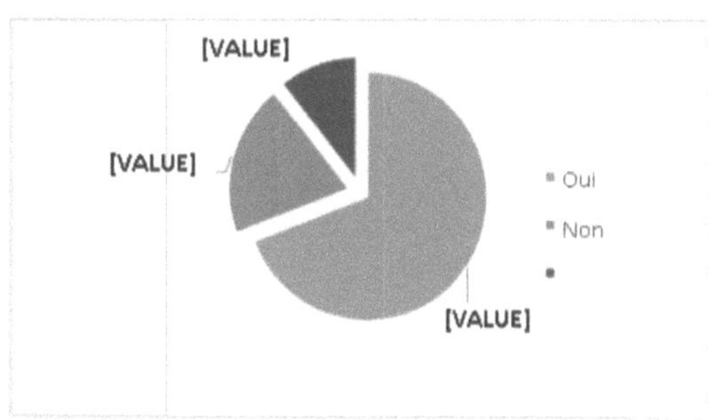

Fig.19 : Nursing knowledge on the entity "Exposure".

- After analyzing the results of different entities on nursing knowledge in primary patient assessment, it was found that 48 of the participants had insufficient knowledge on initial patient assessment according to ABCDE approach and **7.7% had** sufficient level of knowledge(Fig.20).

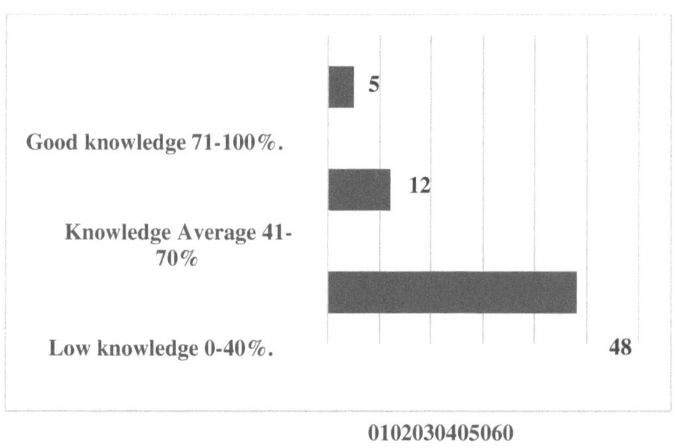

Fig.20: Participants' level of knowledge about the ABCDE approach

IV. The value of implementing the ABCDE approach in the emergency department:

It was found that 44 nurses or 67.7% are interested in implementing this method as a management protocol. (Fig.21)

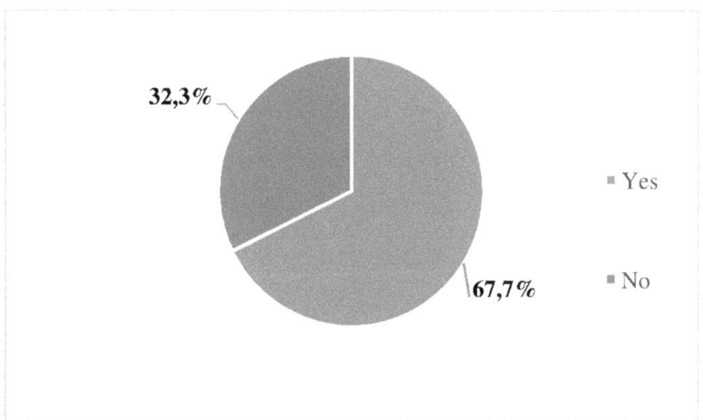

Fig.21 : The interest in applying the ABCDE approach in practice

•   The analysis of the data concluded that 41 of the nurses surveyed (63.1%) were convinced that the implementation of the ABDCE approach in the framework of a protocol within the emergency facilities would improve the quality of practice. (Fig.22)

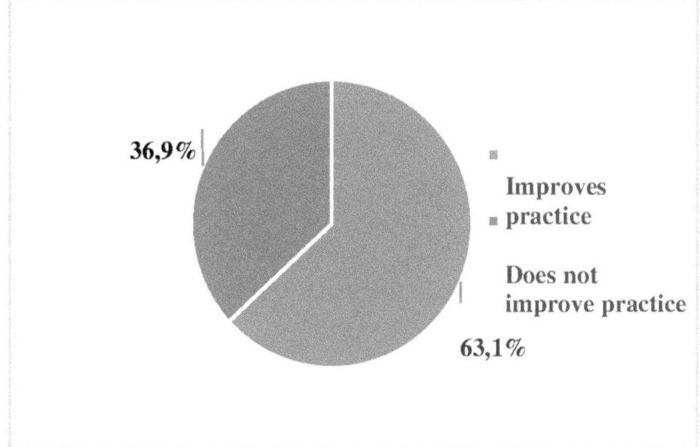

Fig.22: The impact of implementing the ABCDE approach in practice

Discussion

The emergency services constitute a very specific environment, in which we meet situations which put at stake the vital prognosis and situations not foreseen, to guarantee a speed and a continuity of care it is necessary to imply an approach and such a specific protocol which will systematize the work and the assumption of responsibility. We conducted a quantitative descriptive cross-sectional study using a questionnaire among nurses working in the emergency department of Charles Nicole Hospital, Rabta, and Habib Thameur. The limitations of this work were represented by the fact that the time allocated to carry out this work was too limited because of the COVID-19 pandemic, which prevented us from carrying out a larger study. Difficulties inherent to the documentary research: unavailability of works on the scale of Tunisia in connection with the subject of the study, the non collaboration of the nurses in cases, the study led only the theoretical side only on the level of knowledge. The objective of our research work was the evaluation of the knowledge of emergency nurses on the use of the ABCDE approach, and their usefulness in the emergency wards. This study was conducted with 65 nurses working in the emergency department of 3 major hospitals in Tunis (HCN, La Rabta, HT). Thirty-seven (56.9%) were between 30 and 49 years old. The population was characterized by a male predominance (55.4%). Twenty-eight nurses had a seniority of more than 5 years. The analysis of the results of our study showed that forty (61.5%) admitted that the initial management of patients is not protocolized. In terms of the nurses' overall knowledge of the different entities of the ABCDE loop, we found that five nurses had a good knowledge of between 71 and 100%. Regarding the application of the approach in the emergency services, it was found that forty-four (67.7%) are interested in the application of this approach and forty-one (63.1%) think that it will improve the daily practice. In this chapter, we propose a discussion based on the results presented above in relation to the scientific literature, we propose an interpretation of the results that will be divided into four parts.

I. Socio-demographic and professional characteristics of nurses :

From a socio-demographic point of view, our population was predominantly male 55.4%, i.e. a sex ratio of 1.24, with 56.9% being aged between 30 and 49 years. Comparable results were reported in a study conducted in Algeria among emergency nurses, which showed a concordance concerning the gender of the caregivers, 51% of whom were women. It was found that the results were similar in terms of age range between the two studies, with 58.8% being between 30 and 50 years old [4].

More than half of the population studied, i.e. 53.8%, had been practicing their profession for less than 5 years, and 56.9% had been working in emergency departments for less than or equal to 5 years. This youthfulness of the nursing population is explained by the orientation of the Ministry of Health to recruit recently graduated nurses to emergency departments [4].

55.6% of the surveys have already benefited from previous training on emergency care and first aid. A study done in Indonesia in 2015 showed a higher rate, with a more intensified training cycle program so only 17.6% had not received training in the last two years [5].

More than half of the participants questioned working in the emergency room of La Rabta Hospital (55%) had not received any previous training in emergency care and first aid. The lack of interest in training may be the reason for the lack of motivation of nurses to improve their theoretical knowledge. In addition, workload and limited training sessions seemed to be among the causes. One study showed that after simulation-based advanced life support training, the rate of return to spontaneous circulation improved from 58.1 to 86.3%[6]. As well, another study done in England in 2003 assessing nursing knowledge of the initial management of trauma patients before and after a half-day training showed a statistically significant ($P < 0.001$) improvement in the level of knowledge during the post-test[7]. This leads us to insist on the importance of continuous training, even of short duration, given its direct impact on theoretical knowledge.

II. The particularity of an emergency service:

This part is reserved for discussing the results concerning the protocolization of initial management in emergency departments and the impact of the implementation of a management protocol on interpersonal communication

1. Protocolization of initial care in emergency departments :

A predominance that includes 40 staff surveyed (61.5%) reported that care was not protocolized within their services. This may explain the multiple failures of emergency services in Tunisia due to the lack of organization in our hospitals. In France, the nursing protocols of emergency care were set up in 2002, each protocol constitutes a precise medical prescription from the chief physician for a given clinical picture. The firefighter nurse performs a nursing assessment that complements the first aid worker's assessment and implements one of these protocols. The implementation of one of the protocols gives rise to a complementary assessment to the regulating doctor. The service is constantly working to improve efficiency by studying the quality of the intervention: the level of seriousness of the victims, the practical acts and the quality of the care.[8]

Another study carried out over a period of 6 months including 200 polytrauma patients treated by two smur teams in the governorate of Sousè stated that 89.5% of the polytrauma patients had been examined by young doctors in training. Although the intervention guard is not always ensured by a senior doctor who guides the intervention team from a distance, the study showed the presence of missed lesions during the primary assessment contrary to the Ugandan study which includes an evaluation of the primary assessment with less missed lesions by practicing the ATLS approach during the evaluation of the primary assessment and with a presence of the senior doctor during the management. Several actions can contribute to the reduction of these deficiencies in terms of missed lesions during the primary assessment, including the ABCDE approach and the ATLS approach. [9]

2. The impact of implementing a care protocol on interpersonal communication :

Fifty-five of the questioned caregivers (84.6%) affirmed that the implementation of a standardized protocol of management will contribute to the improvement of interpersonal communication and management A comparative study between general practitioners in SAMU of France made by medical students admires our study, Among these GPs who are familiar with the ABCDE(F) algorithm as a primary assessment protocol in emergencies, 67% of GPs in Finistère versus 94% of GPs in Vienne think that this method is a good tool for interpersonal communication in the SAMU, with no statistically significant difference between the two departments [10].

A remarkable majority was for the implementation of a work protocol, as demonstrated by our study in 3 of the major university hospitals in Tunis: Charles Nicole University Hospital, La Rabta Hospital, Habib Thameur Hospital with respective percentages of 85%, 82%, 88%: this indicates the great need for organization of care in our department, particularly the emergency department, and the awareness of the personnel of the importance of a protocol in improving the quality of care.

III. Nursing knowledge of the ABCDE approach:

The analysis of nursing knowledge through this study showed that 63.1% did not know that an approach such as the ABCDE approach exists as a tool for the initial global assessment of the critically ill. Thus, 59 nurses or 90.8% have never used this approach in their practice. According to the article "Initial assessment and treatmentwith the Airway, Breathing, Circulation, Disability, Exposure (ABCDE) approach", published in January 2012, this standardized approach is of easy implementation in daily practice and can be used by all health care professionals [11]. As well as this approach is a currently WHO approved protocol [12].

Results published by T.J. Olgers et al concluded that 83% of emergency department staff used the ABCDE approach in their daily practice [13].

1. Nursing knowledge of the different entities of the ABCDE approach:

• Analysis of the data on knowledge of entity A 'Airway' of the ABCDE loop found that 82% of the nurses questioned recognised that it assessed the risk of upper airway obstruction (UAAO), however 54% did not mention the consequent risk of inhalation in the event of an airway at risk. This result is similar to the study by EriYanuar et al in 2015, conducted on ICU nurses, which showed a rate of participants knowing the same risk of obstruction at 88% [5].

The freedom of the VAS is directly conditioned by a good state of consciousness. Thus 69% of the nurses questioned recognized the risk of obstruction of the VAS following an altered state of consciousness.

• The evaluation of the theoretical knowledge of the participants on entity B "Breathing" of the ABCDE loop, helped us to conclude that 94% related it to the measurement of $SpO2$, 80% to the respiratory rate and 46% to the search for signs of respiratory struggle. These rates were comparable to the results of T.J. Olgers et al where 100% of the participants related this entity to oxygen saturation first [13].

•   Analysis of the results to assess the respondent's knowledge of the ABCDE Circulation loop showed that 97% responded by measuring HR and BP, 80% by palpating the peripheral and central pulses and 55% by checking the color and warmth of the extremities. This rate was comparable to the results of T.J. Olgers et al, where 100% responded by measuring HR and BP first [13].

One of the most important initial assessments of the patient's hemodynamic status is to check the colour and warmth of the extremities. Fifty-five percent of respondents agreed that the extremities should be examined first.

•   Based on the results of the assessment of the participants' theoretical knowledge of the ABCDE loop Disability entity, it was found that 80% responded by performing the GCS examination, 91% by performing the pupil examination and 32% by identifying the signs of localization. This rate was comparable to the result of the study by T.J. Olgers et al, where 98% of the participants responded by doing the GCS score first[13].

•   The analysis of the results to evaluate the knowledge of the respondents on the ABCDE loop entity found that 69.2% answered that it is necessary to perform a skin examination for the critically ill patient, while 20% of the nurses questioned answered that it is not necessary. These results were comparable to the results of the study of T.J. Olgers.al where 92% of the nurses who performed a total body skin examination were found [13].

•   The analysis of the overall theoretical knowledge regarding the ideal initial management of the critical condition patient according to each entity had shown that forty-eight nurses have a low level of knowledge which is between 0 and 40%. According to a study done in Riadh in 2019 it was found that 55.11% of nurses had good theoretical knowledge [14]. As well as another study done in Egypt in 2018 led that 6% had a level of knowledge which is more than 75% i.e. had satisfactory knowledge. [15]

IV.   The value of implementing the ABCDE approach in the emergency department:

In this part of our study we will present the nurses' interest in the use of the ABCDE approach in the emergency room and their implementation as a protocol

1.   The interest in applying the ABCDE approach :

Regarding the interest of the emergency room caregivers in the application of the ABCDE approach as a protocol in initial care, we found that 44 (67.7%) were interested in the application of this method. This predominance indicates such a need for the application of a Protocol that allows for the proper management of care in emergency departments. Among the 33 who responded on the definition of the ABCDE approach we find that 25 (76%) of the respondents answered that it allows for speed in the initial assessment, which results in a high quality of care, This is what is admired by the official site of the fire brigade which reveals that the application of the approach generates an improvement in the quality of the clinical assessment, because of its systematic and dynamic side, like a step forward, on the basis of letters mastered from the youngest age: ABCDE! This systematic and dynamic aspect can also be an appreciable help for the doctor confronted with a serious situation. A homogenization of care, by the simple fact that the language is common between pre-hospital doctors, ISP and first aiders. This common language is concretely translated through our assessment form, with a unique format for the three levels of first aiders, paramedics and doctors. In border areas, interaction is easier with our German and Swiss colleagues, who use this form of assessment. Thus, we are not surprised by the assessments carried out by our neighbours. Moreover, this assessment methodology, which is recognised throughout the world, would enable our rescue workers to integrate without difficulty into an international rescue chain. During the long deployment phase of the method, a form of emulation between trained and untrained first aiders, leading in fine to an overall improvement in practices... [16]

2.   The implementation of the ABCDE approach :

Forty-one of the nurses surveyed (63.1%) thought that the implementation of the ABDCDE approach within the framework of a protocol within the emergency structures would improve the quality of practice.This indicates that the implementation of the approach will be effective, we can confirm our study based on an article of the Swiss Medical Journal on the dechocalisation of polytraumatized patients which indicates that the introduction of such an organized and systematic approach to the polytraumatized patient both in the United States and in Europe has made it possible on the one hand to reduce the number of avoidable deaths to 1-2%, 1,2 and, on the other hand, to improve the outcome of the patient. [17]

V. Study strengths:

This is one of the first studies that was interested in studying the knowledge of nurses on the use of an international approach during their care at the level of emergency services, of the 3 hospitals of the big Tunis.

The study showed the shortcomings found in emergency departments in the management of patients.

VI. Recommendations :

- The overload of work and the lack of staff in the emergency department is
very noticeable
- The importance of involving such a protocol in the initial management of the
patient and not only in the treatment protocols
- Continuous training of emergency nurses to ensure quality care
- The organization of work in emergency departments.

Conclusions

The role of the nurse is paramount in the reception, referral and treatment of these patients in the emergency room and emergency and for a smooth management, the emergency nurse must have the necessary skills to properly manage the critical conditions and emergency situations to give the patient a comprehensive care quickly and effectively.Theoretical and practical knowledge for emergency personnel on patient management is essential and necessary, and it is especially important that emergency personnel are up to date and know the different approaches and protocols for the initial management of patients in critical conditions and use a method that will ensure a rapid but quality management. The ABCDE approach is a powerful clinical tool for the assessment of the primary workup of critical care patients, including pre-hospital first aid, and is extremely helpful in determining the severity of a condition and prioritizing clinical interventions. Of the 65 caregivers surveyed, 55 (84.6%) stated that the implementation of a care protocol will have a positive impact on the collaboration between health care professionals, and therefore the importance of the role of the algorithm in improving the quality of care through optimal assessment. In our prospective study we have been able to highlight unfortunately the insufficiency of theoretical knowledge and practical training of 63.1% nurses and emergency technicians questioned on the ABCDE algorithm and we raise the importance of integrating it within all services except emergency and intensive care services and to improve the knowledge and the level of training of the staff on this protocol which seems well adapted to the current trend of rapid assessment. Our survey also raises the problem of the absence of protocols posted in emergencies, affirming a predominance of 40 personnel among the 65 questioned, so we hope that this study opens the way to the publication of prospective studies of greater scope that will have to study the quality and impact of the protocolization of care as well as to integrate it in the emergency management of patients. The study found that a significant number of health care workers, with a percentage of 63.1%, support the implementation of the ABCDE approach as an effective and beneficial tool to maintain the best possible chain of survival.

Bibliography

[1]-. Reynders S, C Gloeckler, Aymard, Jc. Levraut J. The emergency nurse in Europe. What sorting for the vital emergency: Notion of vital emergency. French society of nurse anesthetists. 2014;7:3-4.

[2]- Smith D, Bowden T. Using the ABCDE approach to assess the deteriorating patient. Nursing Standard:continuingprofessionaldevelopment. 2017; 4:1-10.

[3] :Frederic L.ABCDE, a new approach to emergency department management, 2018;3:2729.

[4] :TOUATI, Fatima.L'infirmier face aux urgences : Les difficultés rencontrées lors d'une prise en charge du patient aux urgences à Tiaret :Les Soins Pré hospitaliers et Gestion des Urgences Vitales :Université Abdelhamid Ibn Badis de Mostaganem.52p,2018

[5] : YANUAR Eri, BUDI Akhmad.The effect of the ABCDE assessment method and an educational session on nursing physical assessment in the general ICU at Dr Sardjito Hospital, Special Region Yogyakarta, Indonesia:a Master of Nursing Science (Intensive Care Nursing)The University Of Adelaide,174p, 2015.

[6] :Amanda KY, Michael JM, Leslie VS, Philip EL, Ryan TM, Colleen ST et al.Use of a simulation-based advanced resuscitation training curriculumImpact on cardiopulmonary resuscitation quality and patient outcomes:Journal of the Intensive Care Society,2019;7:1- 7,.

[7] TIPPET J,Nurses' acquisition and retention of knowledge after trauma trainingAccident and emergency nursing:Accident and Emergency Department, 2003;12:39-46

[8] QUERE, Morgane. Questions to the Chief Medical Officer on emergency medical assistance: When were the PISU set up and what is their use? (online) Sdis29.fr .Consulted on June 25, 2020 ,1p available on internet : http://www.sdis29.fr/a-la-une/882-questions-au-medecin-chef-sur-l-aide-medicale-durgence.html?fbclid=IwAR06p5pO8ksaFh1USC5i4n1eCcqP0D4NaViFPi7RNUFyE3LUqbd9dytCcfk

[9] : OMRI M, BOUAOUINA H , KRAIEM H , CHEBILI N, METHAMEM M, JAOUADI MA. Forgotten injuries in prehospital trauma patients La Tunisie Médicale,2017;Vol 95: 336-340.

[10] MAYET, Céline. La prise en charge des urgences en médecine générale selon l'algorithme ABCDE(F) : Les urgences en Médecine générale : Université de Poitiers Faculté de Médecine et Pharmacie,127p,2018.

[11] : TROELS T,Initial assessment and treatment with the Airway, Breathing, Circulation, Disability, Exposure (ABCDE) approach,2012;5:42-49.

[12] :ATLS France. Surgical Care at the District Hospital. WHO Ed. 2003.

[13] : Olgers T.J , Dijkstra1 R.S , Drost-de Klerck2 A. M, terMaatenJ.C,The ABCDE primary assessment in the emergency department in medically ill patients an observational pilot study: The Netherlands Journal of Medicine,2017;75:106-111

[14] : AMAIRAH F,Assessment of knowledge, attitude and practice regarding oxygen therapy at emergency departments in Riyadh: A cross-sectional study.World J Emerg Med,2017;Vol10:88-99

[15] : MOHAMED M,Nurses' Knowledge, Practices and Barriers Affecting a Safe Administration of Oxygen Therapy:Journal of Nursing and Health Science,2018;Vol7:42-51

[16] WOIS, Guillaume. Towards an evolution of the balance sheet with the

ABCDE: Adaptation took several years,2018;1p.

[17] Schoettker.P ,Blanc .C, Denys .A ,N. Peloponissios. Shock treatment of polytrauma patients, a well orchestrated symphony :Rev Med Suisse,2004;Vol0.23972:59-91.

ANNEXES

Questionnaire

Study of the nurse's knowledge on the use of the ABCDE approach in the management of critically ill patients

This is an **anonymous** questionnaire which is part of a final year project to **study the nurse's knowledge on the use of the ABCDE approach in the management of critically ill patients. Please** respond by checking the box corresponding to the answer that seems most appropriate to you. **Thank you for your valuable collaboration**

I. Identification of the study population :

1-What   is your professional background?

   Multi-skilled nurseEmergency   technician

2-Are you ?

   One ManOne Woman

3-What   is your age range?

20 - 2930 - 4950 years and over

4-How many years have you been in the profession?

   1 year1 to 5 yearsMore than 5 years

5-How many years have you been in the emergency department?

1   year1 to 5 yearsMore than 5 years

6-What   is your role in the emergency department?

   Organizational (unit manager, supervisor, pharmacy manager)

   Nurse at the bedside

7-Have you had any training in emergency care and first aid?

   YesNo

I. The particularity of an emergency service :

8-Is   the management of critically ill patients in your department systematized and protocolized? YesNo

9-Do you think that a prioritized and standardized assessment of care can improve interpersonal communication and care?

YesNo

II. Nursing knowledge on the ABCDE approach

10-Do you know the ABCDE approach :

YesNo

11-Have you ever used?

YesNo

12- Airway : this entity evaluates :

The risk of upper airway obstruction (UAPO).

The risk of inhalation?

Airway at risk in case of impaired consciousness

Intubation is indicated if coma

Neurological condition

VAS free if verbal communication is correct

13- Breathing: what procedures are used to assess respiratory status:

Measuring SpO2

Measuring respiratory rate

Measuring the depth of breathing movements

Measuring heart rate

Look for signs of respiratory struggle

14-Circulation   : How to assess the hemodynamic status of a critical

patient :

Measuring HR and BP

Palpate peripheral and central pulses

Skin recolouring time is >3 seconds

Check the colour and warmth of the extremities

Look for spontaneous turgidity of the jugular veins

15- Disability : what are the examinations to be done for a patient in order to assess the neurological condition :

Glasgow score

Pupil examination

Finger blood glucose

Cerebral radiology

Signs of localization

16- Exposure:Is it necessary to perform a skin examination to assess a critically ill patient: YesNoI don't know

III. The value of implementing the ABCDE approach in the emergency room :

17-Are you   interested in applying this approach in your department: YesNo

18-This   approach :

Allows for rapid initial assessment

Evaluates vital parameters according to the degree of urgency

Follows a certain chronology ?

Is it applicable to all patients?

Can only be used in the emergency room?

I don't know

19-implementation of the ABDCDE approach within the framework of a protocol in the emergency structures :

Improves practiceDoes   not improve practice

Thank you for your cooperation

		Assessment	Management
Step 1	A Airway	• Is The Airway Clear? • Is The Airway Maintained? • Can The Patient Speak? • Are Their Airway Noises? • Is There Air Movement?	• Patient Positioning • Suction / Postural Drainage • Consider Airway Manoeuvres • Consider Airway Adjuncts
Step 2	B Breathing	• Respiration Rate • SpO_2 • Respiration Pattern • Chest Symmetry • Accessory Muscles • Patient Colour	• Patient Positioning • Oxygen Therapy • Assisted Ventilation
Step 3	C Circulation	• Manual Pulse • Blood Pressure • Colour • Capillary Refill Time	• Patient Positioning
Step 4	D Disability	• AVPU • Temperature • Blood Sugar • FAST • Pupils • Pain	• Glucose Supplements • Temperature Management • Pain Management
Step 5	E Expose	• Perform Head to Toe Examination, Front And Back	• Manage Abnormal Findings Appropriately

YOU SHOULD ALWAYS ONLY ASSESS AND TREAT WITHIN YOUR SCOPE OF PRACTICE

AVPU - GCS

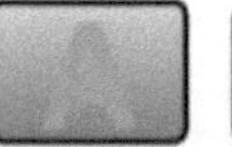 The patient is alert

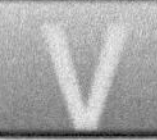 The patient responds to vocal stimulation

 The patient responds to pain

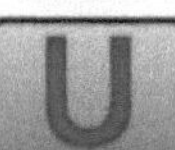 The patient is unresponsive

Glasgow Coma Scale

Behavior	Response	Score
Eye opening response	Spontaneously	4
	To speach	3
	To pain	2
	No response	1
Verbal response	Oriented to time, place & person	5
	Disoriented	4
	Inappropiate words	3
	Incomprehensive sounds	2
	No response	1
Motor response	Normal, obeys commands	6
	Localizes pain	5
	Withdraws from pain	4
	Abnormal flexion (decorticate)	3
	Abnormal extension (decerebrate)	2
	No response	1
Total score	Best response	15
	Threatened airway	≤ 8
	(seek expert help - intubation?)	
	Worst response	3

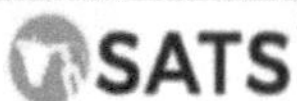 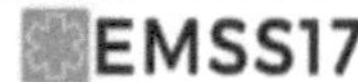

Nørgaard S, Hindborg M, Jensen L, Kristensen C
©SATS Copenhagen 2017 - emss17.sats-kbh.dk **EMSS17**

Summary

Introduction: The use of the ABCDE approach (Airway, Breathing, Circulation, Disability, Exposure) allows a rapid, exhaustive, standardized, hierarchical evaluation according to the level of urgency of the vital distress in the critically ill. **Method**: Quantitative descriptive cross-sectional study which took place with 65 nurses using a questionnaire at the level of emergency services, at the emergency services of the 3 big CHU of Tunis (HCN, Rabta, HT) **Result:** Our study concerned a sample of sex-ratio equal to 1,24. In our results we found that 56.9% of the participants were between 30-49 years old, 55.4% had already received previous training on emergency care and first aid. It was found that 61.5% of the participants stated that they do not have a protocol for initial care, 36.9% know the ABCDE approach and 9.2% have already tried this approach in their practice. In the framework of the implementation of the ABCDE approach 67.7% are interested in the application of the approach and 63.1% think that this approach will improve the practice in the initial care.

Conclusion: Our study has shown that there is little theoretical knowledge regarding the management of patients according to the ABCDE

Key words: ABCDE approach, nursing knowledge, emergency, assessment

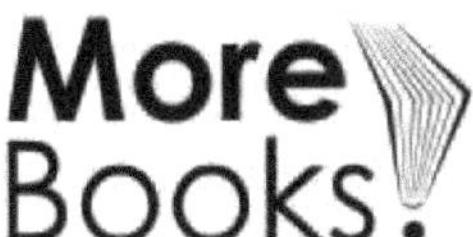

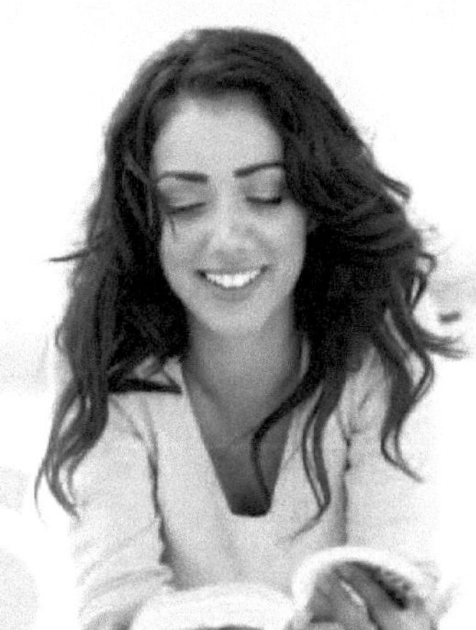

I want morebooks!

Buy your books fast and straightforward online - at one of world's fastest growing online book stores! Environmentally sound due to Print-on-Demand technologies.

Buy your books online at
www.morebooks.shop

Kaufen Sie Ihre Bücher schnell und unkompliziert online – auf einer der am schnellsten wachsenden Buchhandelsplattformen weltweit! Dank Print-On-Demand umwelt- und ressourcenschonend produzi ert.

Bücher schneller online kaufen
www.morebooks.shop

KS OmniScriptum Publishing
Brivibas gatve 197
LV-1039 Riga, Latvia
Telefax: +371 686 204 55

info@omniscriptum.com
www.omniscriptum.com

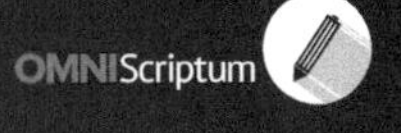

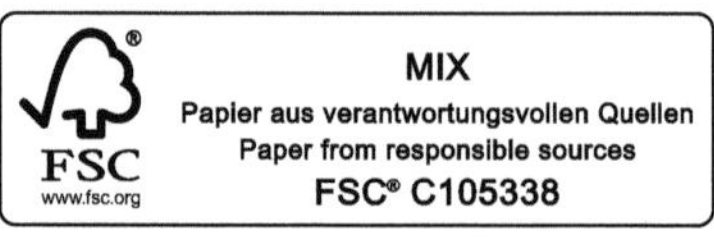

FSC
www.fsc.org

MIX
Papier aus verantwortungsvollen Quellen
Paper from responsible sources
FSC® C105338

Printed by Books on Demand GmbH, Norderstedt / Germany